Straight?
The ultimate guide to understanding DL Men

T L Williamson

Do what your man wants you to do or else someone will do it for you!
—Williamson

Dedication
In memory of my friend Wren,
who passed on way to soon

Credits

Thanks to **Mario Sessions** for his outstanding work on the cover. You are a truly amazing graphics designer. Thanks for your hard work!

Thanks to my amazing friends over the years who inspired me to do this.

Thanks to one amazing brother who means a great deal to me. You know who you are. You'll always be in my heart forever.

Most of all, a special thanks to the men over the years, who were the inspiration for this book.

Words from the Author

I wrote this book as a manual and guide for women and men. Women who have questions or wonder if their man is on the DL. This is for the women whose guts tell them, I think my man is bi-sexual or gay. If you've wondered, then wonder no more. This book will let you know the secrets that men want to hide. I hope from the examples and stories you can begin to question the men whom you date or you are married to. Knowing is much better than wondering and living in the dark. This book is also for men wondering about bi-sexual relationships. This book is for you.

—T Williamson

TABLE OF CONTENTS

CHAPTERS

STORIES

Chapter 1
THE DL PHENOMENON

I guess it was the mid-ninety's and there was a change in the atmosphere. I had just started to realize who I was, or more like, who I was becoming. I honestly really didn't want to accept it. I knew I was gay. I tried to convince myself that i was bi-sexual or whatever, but I couldn't be gay. Gay was bad. Being gay was uncool, or so I thought. I really couldn't grasp who I was. It all stemmed from dating one person who changed my life.

Let's call him Gary. Well, I went to a friend's birthday party in Brooklyn. There were alot of people there including Gary. We were complete opposites. Here I was the conservative, safe black gay man from LI, and he was this thug hood-rat from another part of LI. It was crazy; we met after the party and hit it off. He wasn't my type really, or so my friends would have had me to believe. Gary was a little on the heavy side. I didn't mind this, but one of my shallow friends did.

1

Regardless, we developed a deep loving relationship, which he later only called sex. It was that time that I decided completely cut him out of my life.

We eventually broke up when I got sick of his selfish ways. He only wanted to hookup for sex when it was convenient for him. He had a girlfriend, so I was the second fiddle. I realized this. Point number 1: if you're dating a straight dude or a dude with a girlfriend, know that you will never be the primary. You are just second best to fulfill his needs, when he needs you. That was the case here.

After a year and a half of us being together, we broke up. It really fucked me up bad. I wanted another Gary, badly. I wanted my hood thug dude who would be the same, and I didn't find him right away. Gary was it for me, but I wanted someone to be on the same level as him.

I told that story to show how this all began. Gary was the first of many bi-sexual, dl, and so-called straight dudes that I would meet and chill with over the years. It's funny, but I always looked for dudes, that were like him, that would make me feel like he did. A few came along, but at the end of the day, there wasn't another Gary.

According to Wikipedia, "*Down-low is an African American slang term that refers to a subculture of men who usually identify as heterosexual, but who have sex with men; some avoid sharing this information even if they have female sexual partner(s).*"[1]

Down-low men rarely share information about their sexual preferences. So you think your man is messing around with dudes? Do you think if he was he'd share that information with you? The answer is no. Black men in society are pictured in a certain light.

They're supposed to be manly, strong, sexy and confident. Black women are very critical about homosexuality as well as straight men. Black men that mess around on the "DL" will not tell anyone about what they do. They will not tell their boys, girlfriends, parents or even their closest friends. Later in the book I'll talk about the different types of men that are DL, and how to tell if your man is DL.

Chapter 2
LIVING ON THE LOW

Living on the DL is not easy. You're constantly hiding. You make up lies to cover up other lies you've told. Eventually, you will start to believe those lies as the truth. I know, because I've lived this for many years. I was on the DL for most of my life. It was only in the last couple of years that I decided to do something different. I'm not "**OUT,**" but I'm not hiding either.

To be honest, I met many people in the Gay lifestyle who claimed to be on the DL. It always had different meanings for different people. In the last chapter, we defined it. DL is about living a double lifestyle, period. Back in the day, there was a club in the Bronx for DL bruthas, straight bruthas, and those hiding called "THE WAREHOUSE." It was the staple of the DL Lifestyle in New York City.

Living on the DL has morphed over the years. People still do it more than ever. I think now with the proliferation of Gay Apps (Grindr, Jack'd), Adam4Adam, and even social media, such as Facebook, Tagged and KIK, It's easy for DL men to hook up. I've met straight and married dudes off of Adam4Adam, Facebook, and KIK and other apps.

You will find dudes easily ready to hookup when their girlfriends, wives, or spouses are away. Some of them go as far as specifically stating that, "My wife is away, so I'm looking to play".

While it's not easy for these men (I know), they're always lying and having to hide. This becomes tiresome and annoying after a while, but people do what they must do. Living on the DL means never letting your girlfriend or wife know what you're really doing.

There was a man named Hussein. Hussein was sexy as hell. Chocolate brown-skin shorty. I met him on a website called WBS in the early 90's, it was acquired by Disney in the late 90's and they shutdown the chat room. Chat rooms were popular in the gay community in the early 90's. I met a few dates off that site.

Hussein and I, the first time we met had fooled around. It never quite transpired more to anything than oral sex. I was ok with that. We decided to part ways in 2003 for about four years. He had said something I didn't appreciate, and I wrote him off.

So I reunited with him in 2007, and we became friends again. He came over my house and wanted to erase the computer browser. He was afraid, I would read his email. I'm like, "Dude, what are you trying to hide?" Hussein was clearly hiding. I know he was messing with dudes because we had messed around. He told me about this Latino dude, he had had anal sex with, and the dude was trying to challenge me to fight over Hussein.

I'm too old to be caught up in childish games, so I removed myself from the situation. Hussein in twenty ten proceeded to call me all sorts of names, and talk to me out of my name. I was really done with Hussein, after he verbally assaulted me. His girlfriend had gotten a hold of his phone. I thought he was texting me. Then, I continued to talk to her. I told her the deal about our relations. That's not something I like to or wanted to do, but it had to be done because he was really evil.

After talking to his girlfriend, I was still skeptical. The more I tried to convince her about his infidelity, the more she still didn't want to believe it. I gave her a wealth of information. I think that's how women are. Not my man. Yes! You girlfriend, it's your man. **BELIEVE IT**. He's messing around on you with dudes.

Listen up women, my advice to you is this. *Do what your man wants you to do or else someone will do it for you!* The truth. A man is a creature of sexual urges all bound up inside. Women are emotional creatures. Men are not. You have to enjoy sex, and make it interesting for your husband or partner. If not, someone else will be willing, ready and able. Gay men, get DL dudes because they're willing to fulfill all the man's fantasies and beyond. I'm going to give you a little secret I found out with straight men.

You may not believe this, but straight dudes like their salad tossed. I'm not lying. Yes, there are some that will be like, "Hell No". I found in my experiences, a good majority of them love their salad tossed. They don't want no penis up there, but a tongue or finger (HELL YEAH).

Am I telling you women to do that to your man? HELL NO. There is something about a man with a man that feels organic, raw, exciting and uninhibited. Your man will probably not let you do that, even if you did want to. He admits he doesn't want it done period, but in the bedroom, the tables turn.

Back to the girlfriend. She eventually had to realize the way her man was living with this dude that was kinda suspect. I saw the picture she sent of him, and I said, "YEA HE'S GAY". She knew that already. She knew but didn't want to believe it. Living on the low is meant to deceive you women, but if you believe the lies, then your man will cheat again and again.

Wake up! Don't believe the lies because your man seems like a thug.

One more tip in this chapter. If your man seems overly anti-homophobic, it's probably because he hates himself, and not gay men. The reason is because he's already messing with them or he wants to. Bishop Eddie Long anyone. Well, there are a thousand examples, and we could go on and on. I already know if a man is straight, just by conversing with them. They're not fazed by homosexuals, because they know who they are. If they get hit on, they're simply like, "I don't go that way". They don't start yelling, and want to bash someone's face in, or call them a million names.

Only people with something to hide take the defensive, and want to feel like they're the most masculine men out there. It's a lie. It's a game, and that's what they want you to believe. Don't believe the hype. Women need to question, listen, watch, learn, and believe your gut instinct.

Chapter 3
THE HOMOTHUG

So you got these men who dress up in hip-hop clothing, and fuck with women and men, that's your classic HOMOTHUG.

So in the nineties we saw the dawn of this new breed of gay men. I myself dressed and still do to some degree in hip-hop clothing, as well. I never tried to be a homothug per-say, but found myself liking the hip-hop gear.

The homothug invaded hip-hop and R&B music of the 90's. There were reports of many R&B singers and rappers who were supposedly gay. There clearly was some truth to some of the rumors, but the other rumors were false.

Well if you're wondering if your man is a homothug, then ask yourself the following questions. Does he ever look at dudes in a sexual manner? (WATCH HIS EYES). Has the sex died down in your relationship? Does he have a bromance with a dude? Does he stay over his boy's house alot? Is his boy over your house alot, and are they alone alot?

If the answer is mostly yes, you probably have your answer already. Men who are homothugs have an easy time hiding their male partners than you might think. The woman believe their dude is f***ing a woman and not a man. So thus, it's an easier time in not having to hide their bromantic relationship. Women rarely ever believe their dude is cheating with another man.

This is true even when a male/male friendship seems questionable. If it seems questionable, it probably is. You got to realize as a gay man, this is a great thing. You believe your man is having sex with a woman and never suspect your man is cheating with a gay man. The relationship continues unchallenged because you're looking in all the wrong places. You need to open your eyes and spot the obvious. Pay attention to your man's habits. Bromance's are clearly one step away from romance. Don't ignore your gut instincts. The more you start to question, the more enlightened you become.

Don't accuse without facts. Never. If you do accuse without facts this will cause your man to retreat even-more into hiding. You will not know it. The relationship could end, and now you have zero proof. Rather make it seem like everything's alright, and gather the facts. When you have SOLID proof then you can confront him. You never know what you'll find, if you use a hidden camera in your house.

The homothug's weakness is they feel confident that they can play both sides, and no one will know. They will have a sense of security with the man they are sexing. Never let him know you're on to him. Sometimes it's better to just let the relationship go, instead of staying and being miserable.

Chapter 4
GAY FOR PAY

People that are gay for pay confuse me. I was always interested in how that works. I found out in the last year, just out of curiosity, how any straight man or at least 90% can turn into gay for pay with simple coaching.

What I just said shocked me. I have emails where dudes would f**k for the right price. They admittedly never had sex with a man. So, why would they have sex with a dude? I do know that it's money, that's the reason why. So, they want to still say they're straight.

I'm not buying that. I don't buy that for a lot of reasons. Once you have sex with a dude. It's not the same. If it's a one-time occurrence then OK. If it's something you consistently do, even for money then you're not straight anymore.

Maybe to some degree you're bi-sexual, but it all depends on how much you like it., what act you're doing (TOP OR BOTTOM) and how often you actively partake in it.

There was a gay porn star called SARGE. He did all types of videos from getting penetrated by at least 50 black men over the span of his career and going out being penetrated by a transsexual. He claimed on all the forums that he was absolutely straight. However, he had a video recording of his actions that indicated something totally different.

A source of mine who messed with a gay-for-pay individual before said, "I did mess once with a dude that was Gay for Pay and never understood it. I had to get inside his head. He said he did it because he was stripping first and then was propositioned to do porn, and then porn had led him to doing Gay for Pay. It was an interesting story, and he was an interesting dude. I just didn't understand his story. He was supposedly straight and this girl didn't know, but the internet holds a deep trail. Once you're on, you can't get off.

Most recently I met another Gay for Pay individual, and he has a girl, and is African. He talks to me outside his individual extracurricular activities. He is straight outside of us messing around. He really enjoys it, and never did it before. According to him, he would have no problems fucking a man for money again."

Well, if your man is doing Gay for Pay, you may never know. The only way would be if some man happens to be messy, and reveal his true side-job. Men who are Gay for Pay will always hide their activities and never will tell you what's really going on. They'll make plans to hook up when you're at work, or busy doing something. Watch when they all of a sudden have new clothes, jewelry or money from unknown sources.

The Gay for Pay individual will act like sex is just sex, and it doesn't matter about the gender. They could have sex with a snail and not care. There only motive is to ejaculate.

That being said, an oversexed person will be a prime candidate for a gay-for-pay as they need to be on demand 24-7 and be ready to perform. This type loves the attention and will be hard to catch as they hide tracks very well. They will likely use alternative phone numbers, such as google voice or apps like textnow etc. They will not have messages or texts on their primary phone. Again, it will be harder to catch h them.

Some tips to help you. Check Adam4Adam, Rentboy.com and others. Do a google search for gay male escorts.

Chapter 5
MARRIED MEN

I really could write a whole book on this particular topic. I know so much about this, and probably more than I ever wanted to know. I'm a married man flypaper. I seem to catch them all the time. They seem to be drawn in by me. I don't know why, and wish it weren't so.

The first experience I had was with a man called Tony at the home depot I worked at in my 20's. Tony was a man's man. Sexy as anything and really a particularly attractive man (American Indian, Spanish, Italian mix). We got to know each other at the job, and I was definitely like damn, every-time I saw him. I was at the job, and I heard Tony was in rehab. He had come in for his check, and we exchanged numbers and then one day Tony called me to hang out. I was cool with it. It was after work in the hot summer. Tony had just gotten married. We dropped his wife off at work and went to his crib. We Watched TV. He proceeded to tell me there was something he was curious about. I felt like I already knew what he meant. I tried to pull it out of him and did. He said, "I was curious about sex with a man". We started to go to his bed, and had oral sex.

Afterwards, he talked about moving me in upstairs, and I wasn't interested in doing that. That was crazy. I didn't hear from him, and went a little crazy. He was my first experience. I learned a valuable lesson, don't write a letter to a dude. I did and his wife got a hold of it, it was all over.

So, what I learned with married dudes over time. Keep your mouth shut. No texts, email, letters, etc. Plus, you shouldn't be doing it in the first place. If you are going to do it, trust me it will cause alot of grief. You will always be the second fiddle, and you can never see them when you want to see them. Talk about hiding, everything is hidden, and you really have to be crazy to ever involve yourself with a married dude. I've learned the hard way.

Tony really should have been the last married dude I saw to be honest, but there were two more dudes to come. Both fell in love with me, and me likewise. Rule 2: Don't fall in love with a married dude. It's bad and bring forth nothing but heartache. This should be common sense but I learned the hard way.

Women, if you're married and you think your husband is cheating with a dude, he probably is! Your husband will cheat if he feels like you're not giving him what he needs, or you're not satisfying his urges. I know many married dudes who cheat because their wife is not satisfying them. Women, I know after kids, you're sexual urges go down alot, but you need to take care of your man, or someone else will go and take care of him for you.

Chapter 6
BI-SEXUAL MEN

Bi-Sexual men are supposedly men who love having relations with both women and men. They profess to be open to their partners about their bi-sexuality. With black men, this rarely happens, and not surprisingly so. The black man that is open he will face all types of gay slurs, and derogatory comments. The bi-sexual man has a better chance of honesty, unless he is either married or gay for pay.

Bi-Sexual men love the company of a woman, but desire the sexual chemistry of a man. I dealt with bi-sexual men that had girlfriends before. I even mentioned them earlier in this book.

I've always looked at bi-sexual men in the following way. There are bi-sexual men who are more into women than men, and there are bisexual men who are more into men than women.

In 2002 I met a man called Wayne. Wayne was your sexy bi-sexual brother high-yellow and cute. I really liked Wayne alot. We had a sexual chemistry like no other. Sexually, we just clicked. We were definitely sexual compatible, and had amazing sex every time we connected. Wayne had a girlfriend who didn't know. She was completely unaware of his extra-curricular activities. Well, at least I thought. She actually knew about his trips to the village, and his trips to see me, and other men.

Wayne told me, he was trying to-do the right thing, and we needed to stop having sex. I said, I will support you, in whatever you want. So, I did. Before I knew it, we were having sex again. I finally didn't hear from him. He had moved on, and so I needed to as well, and did.

It was good while it lasted. I realized Wayne was a cheater, and a liar, as most men on the low are. They are manipulative and will stop at nothing to satisfy their needs. You're expendable if you don't serve their agenda. It's all about sex. Women need to understand that. I think sometimes they get it, but other times they think like women. If a woman understood her man, she would be so different with her man. If a woman, understood what it took to please her man, then she would have a method for keeping what's home, home.

Bi-sexual men will always exist. But if you think your man, may be bi-sexual, then ask yourself, what am I doing to keep him? Or is it worth it? Light bulb moment, there are many straight dudes out there...Many. So if your man likes men, then find a man that likes women totally. Simple to me. Difficult for many women to understand. Have a man that loves you and only you. Otherwise, it's not worth it.

Chapter 7
KNOWING YOUR MAN

So you've got this far. You're wondering how I can tell if my man is gay or bisexual. There's no secret formula but there are some suggestions that may help you.

A) **Ask your gay friend** – Well, this could be a good or bad thing. So you suspect your man is sleeping around with dudes. Well, gay men seem to possess this intuition about men in general. Sometimes, they're right and sometimes they're wrong, but a majority of the time they're right. Ask him, what he detects from your boyfriend before you start dating him. You never know if your gay friend will use this to his advantage if your man is very attractive, but you never know. Sometimes an opinion is worth it.

B) **TOYS** - A little unorthodox but see how your man likes stimulation in the back door. He probably will be like heck no, but you never know. If he's kind of down to the idea of the toy, you definitely have a man hiding a secret. Even if he says no, it proves nothing. He probably doesn't want you to think he could be gay or bi-sexual.

C) **Directly Ask** - Telling your boyfriend that you had a fantasy about him, getting blown by another dude, and if he's down for that. He will say no, but indicate that you and another female would do it, at the same time. Building his sexual appetite of two women and potential another sex partner may lead him to be more open to the idea.

D) **Find another straight man** - The easiest way to find out if your man is gay/bi-sexual. Find someone sexy whom you think your boyfriend would like if he was gay. See if this person, can try to propose something to your boyfriend, not immediately, but overtime. If he does bend and wants to-do it, you know.

E) **Watch his patterns** - Cheaters get tripped up in their own lies. All you have to do is sit back, listen and watch. He will trip up somewhere with inconsistencies. It's your job to watch out for his patterns. Does he talk to a man for hours on the phone?

F) **Let it go** - Like I said, women are emotional creatures and as such have a hard time with letting go. You just have to let it go, if you suspect that your spouse or partner is actually cheating. The bottom line is you got to move on. If it's your husband, then you need to figure out what to do. Either way, you need to get out of the situation, before you get hurt.

Chapter 8
GAY MEN

It's easier to get with your man than you think. I've had dudes with females look at me, and so have other gay men. Your man isn't always straight, so you never know what can happen. He can easily exchange his number with a gay man and meet at a more convenient time.

Well, some gay men have boundaries, and others don't. Either way your man is easy prey, especially if he's not getting what he wants out of you. With online websites and apps today you can have instant gratification. You can plan a sex hookup in a matter of minutes. Your man can have sex in your bed before you get home, and act like nothing happened.

Guess what, it happens everyday. Somewhere in the US today, it's already happened and many times. Get used to it. You just need to know how to prevent it.

Never just assume you can leave your man with a Gay Man. Outside your man may display that he hates gay dudes, but then a gay dude is giving him oral sex. You think this really flaming gay man is not a threat. Well, never assume.

You may have a gay friend as your BFF, but they're safe to you, because they're not checking for you, but they're checking for your husband. Or what about the gay barber, or the gay landscaper? Regardless, if you think your man is gay or not, putting them around a gay man is the recipe for disaster.

In finding out if your man is gay or bisexual, you have to monitor his friends. You need to know if they are married or not. Gay or Straight. You do need to pry somewhat in their personal life to protect your man and his future. That doesn't mean going through his phone. Stop it. That's stalker behavior. You just need to pay more attention to his friends that's all.

Your man said, "Honey stay home. It's boy's night out". Maybe it is, and it's innocent, but if you're skeptical, you need to know where they're going. Is it a gay or straight club? Are they hanging out with one boy or their boys? Do you even know?

Common misconception is this, "My man never got f***ed, he's not gay/bisexual." Really? Well, he likes men! It doesn't matter if he was on the receiving end or not. If he's on the receiving end then forget it; he's heavily involved more in the gay lifestyle than he'd care to admit.

Fortunately, most gay men don't want married or straight dudes, but don't mind bi-sexual men for the most part. So if he has the wedding ring, he has fewer options.

Chapter 9
PLEASE YOUR MAN

It's funny that a gay man is telling a woman how to please her man, but I find that most women need help in this department. If this wasn't the case, would you be reading this book right now?

I'll never forget when I was younger, and new to messing around with men, I was at this park in Queens, NY. This guy approached me. He was very attractive and sexy. I was new to this whole man-on-man thing. Anyway, he wanted me to show his girlfriend how to give good oral sex. I was shocked. Why is asking me to do this? Apparently, she didn't give him good head. He also wanted me to give him oral sex in front of other people. I declined.

So, moral of the story is if you won't please your man... someone else will.

A) **Know what your man wants** - If your man wants a massage, then give him the massage. What's wrong with you? If he wants sex, then give it to him. Am I telling you to be his bitch? NO. I'm telling you to act like his partner or wife. Do your wifely part! Not I'm tired. I don't feel like having sex. Depriving your man of sex for months or years, and expecting him to be faithful. You're out of your mind for that type of thinking. He will go somewhere else. I will tell you this. Women have hangups with giving up the goodies.....MEN DON'T. You're husband and a man can be having sex in the next half-hour. Men don't talk. Women do.

B) **CONSISTENCY**- You have sex every two months with your man and he should be faithful. Give me a break. He'll be at my house having sex, and going back to you to go to sleep. Should that get you mad? **HELL YEAH**...do something. If not, then don't complain.

C) **SPICE IT UP**- Men in long term relationships or marriages are bored after years of the same thing. They seek outside interests.

SPICE IT UP. Make sure you try new things. If I'm keeping it different than you, you're man won't be having sex with you anymore, because he'll be having sex with someone that knows what they're doing.

D) **IMPROVE YOUR SKILLS** - If you suck at oral sex, then your man will be getting it elsewhere. Bottom Line. If you practice with him and improve, he'll be staying there instead of going somewhere else. Practice makes perfect. If you don't care, then you might as well end it.

Chapter 10
SEXUALITY

Sexuality is a complex conversation. There really aren't any categories that people somehow magically fit into. I think it's deeper than that. People like what they like. I have found men are just sexual creatures, driven by lust and desires. That doesn't mean every man is some horny machine, but in some cases it does. So let's break down our understanding of different terms we talk about in the book.

1. Straight - Being straight means a man that only has feelings for women, and doesn't have feelings for men. If he does then he will fall under the bisexual category. Straight men aren't afraid to brag about their exploits with women, and conquests. While a majority of straight men have all had thoughts at one point in time of a gay experience, they don't act upon it. If they do act upon it, then they will move down into the next topic.

2. Bisexuality - A majority of the men we talk about in the book are bisexual. The married man, the bi-curious, the gay for pay, and the bi-sexual man fall under this category. Being bisexual means having feelings for both men and woman. Often times, bisexuality can be slanted in one direction or the other. If you sleep with a man, you are bi-sexual period. Most men still want the label of straight, but the straight label doesn't apply here. The problem with bi-sexuality today is that many people label themselves incorrectly as bi-sexual when they're really gay. I always ask a few questions to see the truth. When was the last time you slept with a woman? A few years ago will indicate this person is living as a gay man. If they are actively involved in a bi-sexual lifestyle, we would see them having relations with both sexes. A true bi-sexual will be able to move between men and woman with no issues whatsoever.

3. Gay- Being gay means that you are exclusively interested in the same sex. A bisexual man that actively is involved with woman, can move into the gay category when he demonstrates emotional feelings for a man. It really isn't bi-sexual anymore. Bi-sexual men tend to sex with no strings attached. Gay men get into having a relationship and intimacy. I have known many married men, or gay for pay who become gay, by delving deeper into the gay lifestyle. There definitely is a fine line between bisexuality and gay. Some gay people see only gay or straight, as well as straight people with the same views. There is definitely a clear difference. I believe its emotion based. If you confess love for a gay partner then that crosses the line into the gay category. Sex is still just sex.

Chapter 11
ENDING THE CYCLE

I feel there is a cycle of shame, and self-hate with black men living in a society that doesn't fully accept who they are.

For many years, I was ashamed of who I became or who I was. I felt I wasn't loved. I felt GOD didn't love me, because of who I was. The church told me that I was a sinner, and was going to burn in the lake of fire. People told me this in college, when I hadn't even performed one homosexual act. Did I think about it? Yes, but I hadn't acted upon it yet.

I was confused. How could I turn my back on my creator? How could I fight what I was feeling? I didn't have the answers. I still don't, but I know the war is over in my soul. I love myself. I know God loves me, and I know who I was meant to be, and why God created me! Once you find that out, and begin to love yourself, there really is nothing else that matters, and no one that can bring you down.

I know I mentioned the black community, but this is applicable to all communities. It's not just black men who are engaging in homosexual acts and relationships; it's men of all races and religious beliefs.

My point is this. I will speak from my own vantage point of the black community, but I must say this for all races and groups of people. We need to get better. We need to have a society where we don't judge people, based upon their sexual orientation. That's not an easy thing to accomplish, but it certainly is achievable.

I've been around black women who will berate their man, and call them a faggot or a homo. All the derogative names that hurt. It's no wonder that black men don't tell their spouses. The first reason is humiliation. They know their wife or partner will go and tell everyone they can, to make the woman feel better. Very few women will support their partner and try to make things work, or just peacefully go their separate ways. I admire those women who are examples of what many women are not.

So, you want your man to hide. You want to not know the truth. Hussein's girlfriend that I told you about before, didn't want to know. What about you? Is that easier? Sweep it under the rug. If your man contracted HIV, then you'd want to know. Who was he sleeping with, and why, and how did I catch this? Well, it's too late. You wanted to live in your fantasy world.

Wake up women! This is not a reality show. Even-though, your life may eventually play out like one, you need to get informed. You need to be smarter. You need to know the information so you can be informed. You need to foster an environment where your man could be comfortable telling you the truth.

Let me ask you this. If you knew before you were married, would you have married him? There are plenty of straight men out there for you to marry. Now, you didn't want to know, and he didn't tell you. You have four kids, and he's been messing around on the side. He won't leave you or the kids, but you found out, and your world is upside down. You thought he was a man's man, that's why you married him. Your dreams are dashed now. You can't get a divorce because you need to stay together for the kids. He doesn't want to have sex with you like that, and you don't want to have sex with him either. You feel like your world is falling apart.

There's one cure for these problems. It's one word. It's honesty. Something we don't know about anymore. We throw it out. You forced your man to live on the DL, and now everything he tells you is a lie. Honesty could have eliminated all of this. If only we could tell our partners, and not have fear of being rejected, belittled, embarrassed publicly. If there could be some acceptance, then and only then could couples start to be honest about their sexuality. If you're reading this book, change starts with one person, you. We need to do better. You can do better. Start the change.

CHAPTER 12
TRANSSEXUALS

As I am writing this chapter, what I'm going to write sometimes makes very little sense to me. I do understand it from a thousand foot overview, but personally it doesn't make a lot of sense. You may be wondering the same thing as I'm discussing this chapter, but you really need to absorb what I'm saying, so you don't miss the signs that are clearly in front of you.

Straight men typically do not like to mess with gay men period. It's not there thing. They don't like seeing a man's private parts. It doesn't turn them on in any way, shape, or form. They want to feel like it's a total and complete woman. That really does it for them. As such, you will find that if they're truly straight they tend to gravitate toward transsexuals.

You may be saying, what! Are you serious? I am one hundred percent serious. So, why is this? Well, there are a number of reasons to be honest.

1) **Realness** – Overall, they want the experience to feel as real as possible to that of a woman. This in turn will not diminish their manhood. If I'm doing a chick, or a person that's close to a chick, then I'm not really changing my sexual orientation. I'm still straight. I'm still a man. I'm definitely at this point not a homo, and that's the thing that I want to avoid. I don't want to be labeled anything less than a man.

2) **It's a female** – Well, men that actually go throughout a change to be another sex have to take hormones and injections on a regular basis. They take estrogen shots to make themselves have more feminine features, and as such can easily get rid of the more masculine features. They start to sound and look more like a real women. Those that don't complete the procedure will not be one hundred percent a true transsexual. Straight men want the one that is more realistic. Some men claim they didn't know the difference. Sometimes that may be true, but you really can tell the difference. Sometimes they just don't want to know. Especially, if they have a

so-called "banging chick" they just don't want to ruin the fantasy.

3) SAFE - You can easily hang out with your friends and have this tranny that most people wouldn't really know was, and get away with this easily. However, you cannot do the same thing with a gay man. Your friends would know and you would be humiliated and degraded. It's a safer bet, as a majority of people won't question this as much, where as in the other case they would.

4) ORIENTATION - Well, you don't have to deal with your true orientation, if you mess with a tranny. Deep down inside, you know this is a man, but since she's so feminine, you don't have to acknowledge that fact. It's safe. Later on, the person will have to acknowledge that they are truly becoming bi-sexual, and have those feelings and emotions. It makes it easier to block out those thoughts.

5) SEX - We've addressed this throughout the book. It's easy sex. Tranny's in fact love straight men, because it's a thrill, a challenge, and love the attention. There's so much they have to deal with, that you or I don't have to. If you know your true gender like you probably do, then it makes it easier for you. For the typical tranny they feel like they were born in the wrong body. They feel like the creator made a mistake, and now they feel completely different then their external genitalia. They feel like woman and thus so want to have sex with a man, like a woman would. It becomes a win-win situation since the straight man wants to have someone who is feminine but a woman, and the tranny wants someone who is all man.

The combination here of tranny and straight man becomes the perfect combination here, as the man is in denial of what he truly is orientation wise, and the tranny is also in denial of who they were born to truly be.

I am speaking from my point of view, and if you're a transsexual I'm not saying what you are is wrong. I'm not looking to spark outrage, and have hate mail. I speak as a person who is part of the LGBT community, and it's about acceptance. I accept all members of the community. We may not necessarily agree on everything but I understand. I understand there are different vantage points on sexuality, and I am at a point in my life, where I can accept everyone. I may not agree, but I can accept the person.

Well, my suggestion is this. If either the straight man, tranny, or girlfriend/wife find yourself in a three way triangle. Try and work it out. The straight women will be outraged – "Not my man, and no he didn't." Before you take it there, how about consider talking to your man about his sexuality, and trying to get him to be honest about his feelings. It's a hard thing.

I'm sure many women would just walk away. Walking away to be honest is easier for most people. You can't trust him no anymore. You're going to tell his friends, family, and the Facebook community because you're hurt. He's not being honest, and he can't be honest with you, because you'd never accept it. You should think about that.

He's not like you, because lesbianism is more easily accepted in today's society. A man having any other orientation other than heterosexual is not accepted and to some degree never will. Just because tolerance is preached, doesn't mean it's practiced. I don't think it really is today, or fifty years from now. People are coming out of the closet because they feel in some way it'll be beneficial to them. No one was doing that twenty years ago. Every month you hear a different story now about someone new who has come out of the closet.

Bottom line is this. I'm talking to you straight women. Don't write your spouse or husband or partner off, because you found out that he doesn't fit that perfect ideal of what straight should be to you.

Like I said before, all men think about a sexual act with the same sex at least once in their life. There are many men who are bi-curious. They just need the right person to tip the scales and they can truly bring their thoughts to fruition.

Chapter 13
IS YOUR MAN ON THE DL?

This chapter is probably the most important chapter of the book, but everything has tricks and tips, and you should read the whole book.

So how do you know if your man is messing around? I gave you some tips earlier, but if the book ended there, it would still give you plenty of information, but however I thought you should know how to answer the when and where? So when is he doing these activities and where?

Well, the when is easy. When you're at work, and he's off. When you're asleep, and he sneaks out. When he was late from work, or goes to the supermarket for three hours. What about an extended laundry trip? The gym seems to take a long time to complete every day. You're not stupid. You probably already know the when. You just want to know where. You know why already? To get what you're not already giving him. Well, you think you got the skills, and know he should be satisfied. It's not you ma. It's your man wants something else that you can't give. You can't compete with a male. You don't have the same body parts. You know this. So the why, you already know! You may have deprived him of sex, or even if you've had sex, it's when you want, and not when he wants it. The who, and the why we went over in the last twelve chapters.

Where?

Your House - A lot of men won't necessarily do it at your house, but some will. Right in your face, with absolutely no regard for you or your feelings. This one dude that I messed with called Wayne back in the day. I went to his house once. I had no idea, that it was really his wife's house. He told me his girlfriend and later admitted toward the end of the relationship, that it was his wife. We did it all over hear house. Looking back, it was such a bad idea. I thought about how she must have felt. She felt horrible obviously and I didn't know. There are many dudes out there that don't care about putting it right in your face. In your bed. It's sad.

B) **His House** - He will often sneak out to be with a dude. It's easier and harder to get caught. There is no risk of you coming home earlier, and the bag of worms that situation would open. He can easily have sex, get what he wants and bounce. It's easy for everyone.

C) **HOTEL/MOTEL** - This one is easy to figure out. Guys bring girls to hotels and motels all the time and have sex. It's easy, and convenient and no one really knows about it, unless they're in your room, or see you walking or exiting the hotel together.

SEDIER SIDE OF THINGS

Men want instant gratification and sometimes it becomes harder to have to communicate with a man, just to have sex, so men seek out some instant gratification, which leads us into the seedier side of the gay lifestyle, that many people don't even talk about. No secrets are left unturned here. I'm letting it all out. This way you can find out what your man is really doing in his free time.

ADAM4ADAM- This is one of the websites that has a reputation for meeting men online who are willing to instantly hookup and do whatever you would like to-do. By the way you're man will be an easy target. It's everyman's fantasy for the most part to be with a straight man or bi-curious man. They will be fresh meat on Adam and it won't be long before they are hooking up with dudes on a regular basis. *How do you know if your man is on Adam?* Easy. You could create a profile and see if you can find him. Straight men do not put pictures out there for the world to see. Try again, it'll be much harder for that. Here's the easy solution to see if your man is on Adam. Choose the option that you forgot your password, and have it mailed to your email address. Put his email addresses in, and if it says it's emailing the password well BINGO you know. If it says account not found, then you know, he's not on Adam4Adam. So that's a good thing, right? Yea, it is. However, there are many more options than Adam4Adam. I tried that with Hussein's account and there it was. It emailed a new password request to his account. I knew he was on adam4adam, anyway. Let's find out if your man has been cheating. Were just getting started.

GRINDR - So GrindR is the mobile app version of A4A. You can easily install the app and get quick, anonymous gay sex easily. Its available 24/7, 365 days a year. The thing that makes it really exciting for folks is you get a GPS location that is accurate to 400 ft. or so. With this being said, if your man is traveling, he can find some quick sex easily within feet of him. Maybe someone is staying at the same hotel, or he's traveling around, and takes the app out, and finds some local anonymous action. Although that's how Grindr started out, it really has been replaced by JACK'D for the most part. People still use GrindR, but it's less for quick hookups nowadays and more for people wanting to take things at a slower pace. I guess that all depends on if someone is really horny or not. I've still gotten requests for it, but GRINDR has kind of died off nowadays.

Jack'd - This app was really second to GrindR but has now become extremely popular. Especially with men in the ranges of early 20's to late 30's. Because of the age range that goes on there (GrindR attracts the older crowd) you can easily find a quick hookup. Again, it has GPS location and people can easily send their GPS location, which is accurate and plan on meeting for a quick anonymous NSA (no strings attached) fun. So you're thinking, my man doesn't have those apps? Hmmm....have you checked his phone. There are many more examples of gay apps such as Growlr (for heavyset men), Guy-spy, gay.com, and although not gay websites, people use Tagged, Facebook, and Twitter to make hookups as well. So, your man may not have gay apps, but you don't know if his Twitter, Facebook, and Tagged are just innocent or something that'd shock you.

The Old Fashioned Way

Do you really think that people in the 1960's had Jack'd, A4A, etc. They didn't. They still had crazy sex in crazy places. So how did they do it? It's still being done.

Bathhouses/Saunas- This has always been popular in the gay community as a way to hookup, and get satisfied quickly. Typically, you don't see a lot of straight men at bathhouses but it does happen. People still go. Gay men are still there, and they still are in business. Most straight men are nervous to go here, but many straight men have. It's good to know about, but your man will not likely go here.

PARKS - You are much more likely to see straight men here. It happens all the time. It's nearby, convenient, and you can get out real quick. Do something in minutes, and bounce. I know a married dude who use to frequent Prospect Park in Brooklyn, NY. Most large parks have a gay section and on a hot summer night, they come out in droves. Another example in NY is central park. Buried deep in the park is an area where gay men and straight men come and do their thing and bounce. It's easy and you will definitely like I said, find many straight men in the parks.

Movie Theaters - Another place that straight men frequent is the XXX movie theaters all over the country. Again, it's easy to get a quick blow job or possibly have some penetration sex, and then get out and go back to their wife and kids. No one will be the wiser to it. The only problem is actually going into the movie theatre, because sometimes these theaters are located in public areas. That could be a problem but usually the men go at night, and hide their faces. They're usually open all day sometimes, and your man will make a pitstop and keep it moving. You're none the wiser to it.

SEX PARTIES - Yes again, you will often see amongs the many gay men, some straight men up in the mix. It's again, quick, easy sex, and they can go and mess with multiple partners, get off and bounce and go back home to wifey. They usually occur on weekends, and special holidays. Every major city has some event happening every week. You never know if your man, will find his way to one of these. Hopefully he's using a condom at these events.

GLORYHOLES - Another typical one that you will find your DL man attending are these glory holes that people have. It's an easy way to have anonymous quick sex, with not much thought involved. They can go in, and get their dick sucked and bounce like nothing ever happened. It's happening every-day. Craigslist is the way that many of these men advertise stuff like that. Your man may do this and you'll never know. I don't recommend that women check your man's browsing history, but if you're the crazy type. I guess it never hurts☺.

I wanted to make it clear, that this stuff is happening every-day. You don't know when. When you're at work or on his way home, it could potentially happen any-time. Do your research. If he has a gay app on his phone, he wasn't doing research. You're not dumb. You have all you need to know.

Chapter 14
LIVING IN FEAR

I titled this chapter "Living in Fear" for a reason. When you live with someone, who you suspect is living life on the DL, there is some inherent fear.

The biggest fear for women is what he is bringing home to me. I spoke with one of the women that was the wife of the DL guy I dated. She said, she would not have sex with him, because she feared, she would contract something. HIV is no joke. Your life is in jeopardy. If your man is clearly engaging in homosexual acts, then you need to get checked out now. Don't wait. Do it now. You need to know.

Don't wait for mounds of evidence, when the evidence that you need is starring you in the face. Get help. Get out, and get tested. You can't live with the fear of what if he's doing xyz. If you strongly feel that, then it's probably the case. He probably is doing those things that you think. The only question left is how long are you going to deal with it, or do you want to deal with that. I know one couple that was very honest. The man told his wife about his sexuality and that they couldn't marry unless she accepted it. She did. He did his thing, and so did she. They made that pact. I actually really admired them. It takes courage to come clean.

To be honest and say hey this is who I am. If we hide, we keep falling into a deeper abyss of not being honest. It starts with one person. If you're a straight man and reading my book, have the courage to tell your partner. If she is immature and does things to make you humiliated and degraded, It will come back to her. If you know you got a ghetto girl, then obviously don't tell her. If you have a loving and open intelligent black woman, then certainly tell her.

The more we let go of secrets and can be honest, the more we can heal, and start to come out of the closet of our lives. People are

DL, because they feel society puts them into the closet. Maybe that is true to some degree. I feel we put our own-selves into the closet. I think it's time to come out the closet, and LIVE OUT LOUD.

Story #1:
THE HOMOTHUG

It was 1998, and the relation I had with Gary had deteriorated. I was ready for change. I had a party and my best friend invited his friend over. We'll call him Tony. Tony was similar to Gary with that little thug appeal. I was clearly looking for that, so I got hooked easily.

I had way too many drinks that night. I was dating someone at the time. Even so, I was drawn in by this dude called Tony. We were flirting all night, and at one point he went into the bathroom, and I followed him in, and we kissed. It was kind of hot. Anyway, I found out Tony had a common-law wife and kids. That was messed up, and he was at a gay party. That whole thing I think attracted me even more to him.

We exchanged numbers at the end of the night, and the next day he came over. We had sex, even-though it was wrong, and crazy. I guess I didn't mind it. We hung out and eventually became cool friends, but I was no longer sexually attracted to him.

So we hung out, and we were chillin alot. He spent a week over my house, and it was purely innocent. We moved on. A friend of my best friend came up, and was hanging out. He met Tony, and we went out to the club. We came back, and they were staying over. Anyway, Tony was f***ing my best friend's friend on the living room floor which was tacky.

After that we still remained friends and hung out. I learned he had issues with me for whatever reason. He would try and tell other people about our sexual experiences at different places we went. I never knew why. Even in front of alot of people, he would just verbally attack me. I think deep down, he still really wanted to be with me. I don't know why he wanted me. I had moved on. I haven't heard from him since 2003, and neither has my best friend. I think he may have just tried to deal with his family.

I hope that's the case. He was at least a real HOMOTHUG. Attending gay clubs, and going out to gay events is not really cool, especially when you have a wife and kids at home. I really think Tony has at least if temporarily left his HOMOTHUG past, and began to be the father and husband he should have been.

Story #2:
GAY FOR PAY?
(CONTRIBUTED STORY BY ANONYMOUS)

I don't know. I have an affinity for straight men. It's so much different from being with a gay man. It just feels different. So I put up an ad, and I met this sexy black African dude. He never had an experience before with a dude, and you can easily tell when someone lies. He's just a freak who likes sex.

He's in the military and his name is Manny. Manny is really attractive. Every time I was with Manny it felt really good. I tried to push the limitations with him as far as what we could do. He let me actually lick his hole one-time and seemed to enjoy it alot. I couldn't believe how much it turned me on, what a freak.

He would communicate with me afterwards. I never understood why. This is an arrangement right? It's not a friendship, and we aren't cool peeps. Were two people that seem to get together and have sex. I give you some dough and you bounce right.

It's supposed to be simple and cut and dry. Not complicated. Anyway he likes to talk to me about how big his dick is, and how I like it. He send me his photo of his dick, and see what I'm missing. I think he really just likes having women and men after him. The second part is since his first experience with me, he contacts me, and not really the opposite that much.

He knows how he likes to be pleased and likes the fact that I can pleasure him. He's definitely a freak and as a freak, enjoys just getting off. He's interesting. I just wonder how he could easily go from being straight to a gay-for-pay relationship at the turn of a light switch, effectively becoming bi-sexual.

Well, my comments to this story are this; I think that manny really wants money and since he's a freak, doesn't really care whom he sticks his thing into. He's not thinking this will make me bi-sexual or this will make me Gay. It's all about the money, and that motivates him.

I really believe most straight or bi-curious men will do something at the drop of a dime, if there is monetary involvement. They will be cool with having sex with a man, if it means paying the light-bill, or needing some new sneakers, or just being able to have some extra money. Money really talks, and the gay-for-pay individual is all about what I can get out of this. It doesn't matter if they get sexual gratification as long as they are satisfied.

Manny seems different. It seems he really does enjoy the sex, and outside of that he really enjoyed the writer. He's interested in some deeper meaning with the gay guy, but doesn't quite know yet, what he wants this to be. Only time will tell.

Frequently Asked Questions

Q: I feel my man might be cheating on me with another man. He and his good friend who are gay have a bromance so what do I do?

A: I want you to listen to your gut. What does it tell you? It could be simple as a bromance, but if his friend is gay, and openly, then it could give them the opportunity to try something in the future. Accusations could actually push him to his gay friend, more than break the two up. I recommend that you monitor the situation. If sexual patterns change then there might be something to worry about. It doesn't mean necessarily with the gay man, but he could be cheating with someone else.

Q: In the book you talked about transsexuals, and the possibility of my man potentially fooling around with one. Will he also fool around with gay men?

A: I'm happy that you asked the question, and I will further explain something I left out in the chapters. Your man most likely may have sex with a transsexual, but it's not one-hundred percent guaranteed. What's more likely is that he will have a potential relationship of some sort with a straight/bi-sexual man like himself. Why? Because men who are married, want someone like themselves. It gets less messy that way. They don't want a tranny or a gay dude blowing up their spot. It's simpler and easier to find a man who has kids and a family. This way there's no pressures, and they both can have sex when it's convenient. I've seen this happen many times. They will just completely disregard gay men.

Q: You talked about different websites that potentially my man could use, and I can check them to see if he's on. Do you recommend I check all of them?

A: If you have a reason to check them, then do it. If you don't, then you should just trust your man until he starts to lie constantly. It's easy to tell because he will tell lies to cover more lies, and continue the process about everything.

Q: My man acts very effeminate. Does this mean he's gay?

A: There is a thing called metrosexual. Some dudes are just like dat. They seem gay but are not really gay. They're soft but not really gay. It happens. I don't think you should assume anything until your man, gives you reason to believe such. Now, I involved myself with someone who was very metrosexual and straight, but since we fooled around a couple times, and he liked it, and wanted more. He would take the bi-sexual category now. Oh well, so yes someone can change to enter the DL lifestyle. I think you just need to make sure their effeminate ways, don't confuse you into thinking they are actually something completely different.

Q: If my man tells me, he's attracted to men and wants to pursue a bi-sexual relationship, what do I do?

A: If you find a man like that, you should really try and find out about salvaging that relationship. A good man would tell you the truth like this, unfortunately men do not. If he's interested in relations with men. How do you feel about that? Is that something you can handle? If not, and there's nothing wrong with saying no, then you should both discuss it. Plan on making a separation if that's what's needed. Otherwise some therapy may be a good option. You can both figure out, what bothers you, and what you need to work on.

CONCLUSION

Women love to say that men are dogs, and at the same time do nothing to keep their man. The problem is that you gave up a long time ago. You aren't ready to do what it takes to salvage your relationship. If you were, no man could come between that. The man will always choose his wife and family over another dude, period. Hands Down. So instead of complaining, do something.

I wrote this book because I got tired of hearing women's sob stories and what women aren't doing. This is to educate you and save marriages and families. The Family Pride Coalition has recently estimated through their studies that at least 20 percent of all gay men in America are in heterosexual marriages. We must wake up. This doesn't include bi-sexual men, and isn't one-hundred percent accurate. I believe the number is much higher. If we included bi-sexual men the whole number increases.

Women are the ones who will contract HIV/AIDS. Women are the ones whose lives and families will be destroyed. Women are the ones who will need therapy and counseling because of something that could have probably be avoided.

Don't get me wrong, there are gay men hiding in relationships who are gay period. Working on the relationship won't change their feelings. Homosexuality is genetic. Some people say its learned behavior, but no one wakes up and says hey, "I want to be gay or this is who I want to be." Being gay is not a choice, but I will not debate this here. I will say regardless women need to respect men better, and understand their man. Understand what they feel, and go through. Understand the man's needs, and respond.

We can be better. We can keep families and relationships together, by creating a unity of trust in our relationships. Men should be able to voice how they feel about their sexuality without judgment, and woman should respect here man's views

Mutual respect is what it takes. We certainly won't erase bi-sexuality at all. We certainly can make it easier for our men to feel comfortable with who they are, without fear of repercussions. I hope that you will gain some insight and help from this book.

Straight? My answer is that is still up for interpretation.

Sincerely,

T L Williamson

SOURCES

"Down-low." *Wikipedia*. Wikimedia Foundation, 24
May 2014. Web. 24 May 2014.